Sugar Detox

Total Healthy Body Makeover

By Katie Lenhart
Copyright © 2013

Income Disclaimer

This book contains business strategies, marketing methods and other business advice that, regardless of my own results and experience, may not produce the same results (or any results) for you. I make absolutely no guarantee, expressed or implied, that by following the advice below you will make any money or improve current profits, as there are several factors and variables that come into play regarding any given business.

Primarily, results will depend on the nature of the product or business model, the conditions of the marketplace, the experience of the individual, and situations and elements that are beyond your control.

As with any business endeavor, you assume all risk related to investment and money based on your own discretion and at your own potential expense.

Liability Disclaimer

By reading this book, you assume all risks associated with using the advice given below, with a full understanding that you, solely, are responsible for anything that may occur as a result of putting this information into action in any way, and regardless of your interpretation of the advice.

You further agree that our company cannot be held responsible in any way for the success or failure of your business as a result of the information presented in this book. It is your responsibility to conduct your own due diligence regarding the safe and successful operation of your business if you intend to apply any of our information in any way to your business operations.

Terms of Use

You are given a non-transferable, "personal use" license to this book. You cannot distribute it or share it with other individuals.

Also, there are no resale rights or private label rights granted when purchasing this book. In other words, it's for your own personal use only.

Sugar Detox

Total Healthy Body Makeover

By Katie Lenhart

Table of Contents

The Beginning

A hundred years ago you would have had about 15 grams of sugar per day, primarily simple sugars, found in fruits, vegetables and milk products. Today, studies show the average person gets up to 125 grams of fructose per day. It's not that fructose is dangerous for you in moderation. Too much of anything just isn't a good thing.

Why are large amounts of fructose harmful?
* Breaking down fructose is extremely taxing on the liver
* Over dosing on fructose manifests negative effects on the body overall, evident in the crazy amount of soda we consume in general.

Sugar is something most associated with sweet and tasty. We use it to explain why something tastes sweet. If we don't like the taste of a bland flavor of tea we might sweeten it with sugar, honey, raw sugar or sweetener, in order to enjoy this beverage. If a tomato sauce is too tart, all you have to do is add a few tablespoons of sugar to hit the jackpot.

We live in a world that revolves around sugar and knowingly or not this screws our health and happiness, emotionally, physically, mentally and socially by overdoing it with sweetness. When we lose our job or get dumped by our boyfriend we'll temporarily sooth our sadness by overloading our system with sugar. This will boost our mood artificially by spiking our blood sugar levels dangerously high, allowing us to "think" we're feeling better. However this short-lived sugar high induced by bags of candy, tubs of ice cream, pastries, cookies and other sinful delights, ends as quickly as it began and your energy levels will plummet straight down to the bottom of the barrel, often, triggering depression, a sense of shame, uselessness and overall negativity. Just not a place anybody wants to be.

Sugar will take your natural negative emotion and manifest it, leaving you feeling worse than worse and poisoning your body to boot.

Sugar Bug - In 2011 the global production of sugar was about 170 million tons. The average person eats up to 30 kg of sugar every year, about 300 food calories each day per person. That's a heck of a lot of extra calories with zero nutrition!

The sad thing is you actually teach yourself to crave sugar. If you are truly hungry and grab a candy bar or muffin to curb your hunger until dinner, you are literally programming your body to want sugar whenever you are hungry. If you make a point of making healthy food choices when your body is signaling to you it needs refueling, then you won't be craving sugary sweets continuously. Good to know.

Time for us to figure out everything you need to know about sugar so you can decide if Sugar Detox is the right move for you and your long-term good health and happiness.

Sweeteners, Natural and Refined Sugar

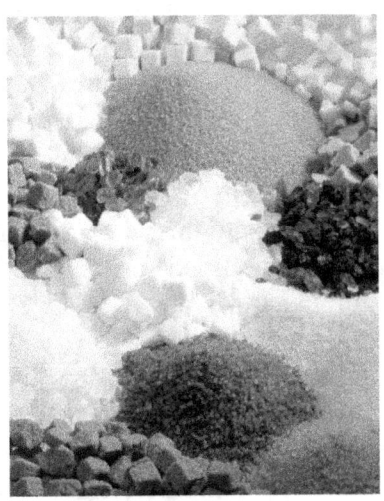

What is Sugar?
It's the generalized name for a group of chemically-related substances that are sweet in flavor, many which are used for food. Looking into the scientific makeup, sugars are carbohydrates. This means they are made of carbon, hydrogen and oxygen. There are different kinds of sugars:
* Simple Sugars
* Granulated or Refined Sugars
* Chemical Sugars or Sweeteners

Simple Sugars - Are often called monosaccharide's. They include glucose, galactose and fructose. Simple sugars are quickly absorbed into your system for energy, having just one or two units of sugar. They are found naturally in foods, but can also be present in processed choices. Natural food examples are vegetables, fruits, milk and milk products. These food choices are loaded with essential vitamins, minerals, and protective antioxidants, making them healthier than processed or "fake" foods.

Simple sugars are present in the tissues of plants, but not in large enough quantities to extract. Sugar cane and sugar beet are the exceptions to the rule here. Sugar cane is a tropical grass that sugar is extracted from. Sugar beet is cultivated and collected is cooler climates. It's a root crop.

Refined Sugars - Table or granulated sugar usually used as food is sucrose. It's a disaccharide like maltose and lactose. We don't need to get too deep into this, but it is important to not some health experts agree refined sugars are more dangerous than unhealthy saturated and Trans fats.

Other Refined Sugars are . . .
Sanding Sugar: It's more coarse than regular granulated sugar, which makes it great for decorating desserts, adding to cold desserts to make sweet without interfering with the desired texture.

Powdered Sugar: You may know this one as confectioner's sugar, what you might sprinkle over cookies or on your French toast or pancakes. This is the smoothest version of refined sugars.

Super-Refined Sugars: These are typically used in commercial foods, things sugar loaded beverages, soda, and meringues.

Sweeteners - These are sugars that have been altered chemically. Technically they aren't classified as sugars, but are thought to be and often substituted for sugar. These "fake" sugars are used to make food lower in calories.

Do we need sugar to be healthy? Yes.

FACT - We can get all the sugar our body needs through natural or simple sugars. Refined sugars are only going to add extra nutrition-less calories to your diet. Increasing obesity and the risk for serious disease like diabetes, while stressing out your digestive processes and interfering with the absorption of vital nutrients.

My Thoughts . . .
Understanding the differences between these three main sugars is important in recognizing where and if they fit into your diet. Experts agree our society is overloaded with unnatural sugars that are dangerously addictive and deadly over time. Learning how to remove these harmful sugars is going to take one step closer to a healthier happier optimal you.

Sugar and Body Function

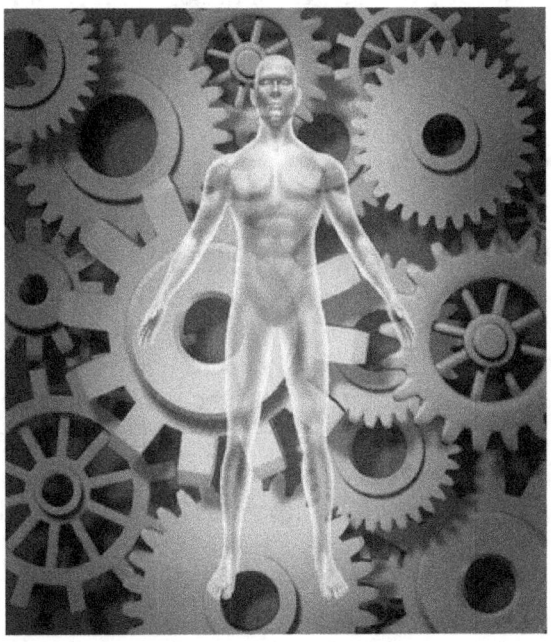

Glucose is used by the body metabolism to give you energy to execute activities, the primary function of sugar. It can also be stored as energy and helps with preserving your lean muscle mass.

Here's the basics of how sugars break down in your system
Large molecules of glucose are found in the starches you eat. It's your digestive juices that break starch down and pull out the glucose. The glucose and various other simple sugars you eat will travel through your small intestine into your bloodstream, and with the aid of insulin, they transfer into your liver subsequent tissues. Now these sugar molecules are ready to fuel your system or be transformed into various kinds of physiological molecules.

15

Sugar Body Functions Are:

Fuel - As mentioned previous your body uses the energy from sugar for your cells. Through glycolysis cells oxidize glucose to make lactate or pyruvate. It continues to metabolize into ATP, adenosine triphosphate, a molecule known for very high energy that gives your cells energy for such actions as muscle contraction. Your body also gets energy from fructose (fruit/table sugar), and galactose (milk sugar). When calculating calories consumed, sugars account for 4 calories per gram.

Saves Protein - With choice your body naturally opts to use complex carbohydrates for energy first, then proteins and fat. However if you don't fuel your system with enough natural sugar it will opt to use protein as its number one source of energy. When your system isn't getting enough sugar you will burn up the amino acids from proteins which normally give energy to your system. If this happens the protein you eat isn't available for other uses including muscle building or keeping your muscles firm and strong. Making sure you are giving your body enough "good" carbohydrates to function is going to help ensure you don't eat away your smooth and powerful lean muscle mass.

Sugar Bug - Muscle burns more calories than fat, helps you remove pesky aches and pains, avoid injury and illness and contributes to a better quality of life. Important to note is people of any age and even those in poor health can build lean muscle mass. Experts agree the body never stops having the ability to build lean muscle. No excuses, where there's a will there's a way.

Stores Energy - It doesn't matter what you are eating because if you consume more than your body needs it will convert it into fat. Excess sugars are transformed in glycogen, stored as starch that your liver and muscles hold for later use. Your muscles use the muscle glycogen, but glycogen of the liver is universally available to other tissues. This stored glycogen has a low threshold. This energy source is critical because your brain needs it. If your blood sugar levels happen to be low, glycogen is required for brain function. Perhaps this explains why it seems harder to concentrate when your energy levels are down?

Other - Extra sugars can also be transformed into fatty acids or amino acids. Depending on how your body functions as a whole, you may end up storing excess sugars from carbohydrates into fat tissue.

My Thoughts . . .
Sugar is a key component in overall good health. It's necessary to support optimal energy supplies for daily function in supporting muscle growth, brain function and extra energy. Serious issues arise when specific sugars, refined and/or chemical sugars are used in excess and directly interfere in smooth body function.

Sugar Dangers to Your Health

Brain and Thinking
New research shows having high blood sugar levels may impair thinking. People with high sugar intake responded slower, were less accurate in mathematical problems, and had slower mental recollection overall.

Immune System Function
Unfortunately sugar has a negative impact on immune system function. White blood cells help protect your body from disease. Unfortunately, your body essentially views Vitamin C and sugar as the same. So if you are eating loads of sugar your cells are absorbing sugar instead of Vitamin C and this will compromise the health and effectiveness of your immune system.

Addictive Tendencies

Sugar is one of those substances that is extremely addictive, partially because it's so quickly and easily absorbed into your bloodstream and provides immediate energy, although short-lived.

Obesity
We all know that sugary foods are loaded with extra fat and calories. These are substances often foreign to the body, items it just doesn't need, yet we continue to fill our bodies full of all of these unhealthy, nutrient-less, sugar laden sweets continuously. It doesn't matter what type of food you are eating. If you eat more calories than you are burning or your body requires you are going to get fat. In our technologically savvy and often automated society, just a nice way of saying "lazy." we hardly burn enough energy to keep our weight stable by eating healthy.

Too much sugar directly contributes to obesity and on the way to reverse the situation is to ditch the sugar, or at least start by reducing it considerably. Makes sense right?

My Thoughts . . .
Removing substances that interfere with good health or jeopardize good health need to be removed. You are important and so is your health, mentally, physically, emotionally and socially. Sugar in excess, particularly refined sugars make people fat and miserable, interfere with a clear head and can make issue with the health of your immune system. Sugar Detox is going to breathe new life for you if you want it.

Reasons to Avoid Sugar

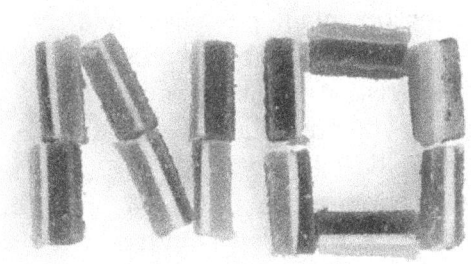

* Steals minerals from your body
* Causal factor in heart problems
* Contributes to cancer
* Triggers and supports premature aging
* Steals energy
* Triggers unhealthy cravings
* Causes obesity
* Linked to diabetes
* Player in causing osteoporosis
* Instigates various skin conditions including eczema
* Causes arthritis and other circulatory issues
* Robs essential minerals from your system
* Tips your blood acidic
* Destroys teeth
* Negatively affects blood sugar levels
* May cause gallstones and ulcers
* Takes the wind out of your immune system function
* Stresses vision
* Lowers blood sugar levels
* May cause hyperactivity, depression and anxiety

* Can damage kidneys
* Narrows blood vessels restricting blood flow
* Leads to alcoholism and other substance abuse
* May cause appendicitis
* Can cause nasty varicose veins
* Can decrease glucose tolerance which can trigger diabetes
* Causal factor for toxemia in pregnancy and eczema in kids
* Triggers headaches and high blood pressure
* May increase the risk of Alzheimer's
* Fools negatively with your digestive system
* Can stress the capillary lining
* Interferes with clear thinking
* Stresses memory and overall system function
* Causes bloating and irritability
* May cause hormone imbalance
* Can interfere with genetic makeup
* Causal factor for cataracts

My Thoughts . . .
It's pretty obvious sugar in excess is only going exaggerate any health issues you have, mental or physical. What many don't recognize is that sugar in excess can seriously kill you! By interfering with the finely tuned system you have, blockages are created and this will directly harm your health. You are in charge of you. If you want to make the changes necessary to steer clear of preventable disease and feel better about yourself in the process, take the time to get rid of the sugar, you don't need and just make room for the stuff you need.

Sugar Tidbit - What You Need to Know About Sugar and Drinks - It's not just foods with sugar in them that are causing issue with our health today. Many drinks are loaded with sugars that contribute to causing your body harm while making you "think" you aren't really doing anything wrong. Sports drinks, sodas, energy drinks, fruit juices and sweetened teas are large contributors to our sugar problem. Here

are a few beverage sugar facts that are going to knock you on your butt.

* One can of soda has about 65 grams of sugar or 22 packets.
* In order for a ten year-old to burn the extra calories from a can of soda they have to bike hard for at least 30 minutes.
* An adult has to walk fast for an hour to burn off a can of soda.
Check the ingredient list on your beverage. If you see the following it is likely LOADED with sugar. Opt for water, herbal tea or clear soup instead.
- corn syrup
- fructose or fruit juice concentrates
- sugar or honey
- sucrose or dextrose
Believe it or not, beverages in excess do contribute to fat gain and serious health issues over time.
Tips for Smart Drinking
* Skip the high-calories sugar loaded drinks
* Add lemon, line and other herbs and fruit to make water dazzle
* Always have bottled water available to grab
* If you MUST have a beverage with sugar opt for the smallest size

Sugar and Disease

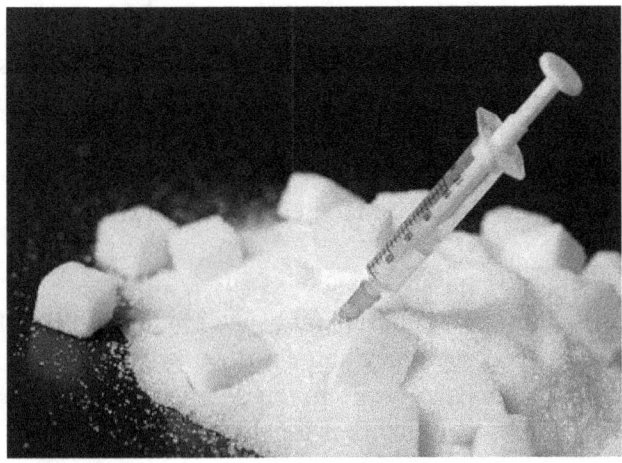

It's all about prevention. If we can change our learned eating habits with reasonable actions to help prevent serious disease and heartache, literally, down the road, isn't it worth the effort?

This all starts with being aware of our options. What causes disease and what we can do about avoiding or more realistically reducing our negative action, some is better than nothing right?

Understanding it's usually not one action or one item you are eating that's going to cause your health to plummet. Most are multi-factorial and all interdependent either on the surface or beneath. I'm sure there are zillions of foods we eat and lifestyle choices we make that trigger disease and illness that we, including medical experts, know nothing about. The best plan of action is to gather information and use it where we see fit to help us better our quality and quantity of life.

Here are a few diseases scientists have directly linked to sugar.

Diabetes
Diabetes is also called diabetes mellitus. It's a bunch of metabolic diseases where you have high blood sugars, because of not enough insulin production or your body cells aren't reacting as they should, sometimes both. If you have high blood sugar you will probably pee a lot (polyuria) and be really hungry and thirsty, polyphagia and polydispsia respectively.

There are 3 main types of diabetes, Type 1, Type 2 and Gestational.

Diabetes is often preventable and caused by unhealthy life habits. Not exercising regularly and eating poorly doesn't help any. Genetics also plays a key role in the development of this disease. This metabolism disorder for the most part can be prevented, which is great news.

So where does sugar come into the picture and how?
Sugar gives your body extra calories and is easily absorbed. This means the more sugar to consume that greater the risk for diabetes, Type 2. It doesn't take much either. Experts agree that just one "sugary" beverage more per day will more than double your risk - yikes!

Cardiovascular Disease
Cardiovascular Disease is also known as blood vessel and heart disease. It includes many problems, most of which include atherosclerosis, a condition which is a result of the buildup of plaque in your artery walls. This causes your artery passages to narrow and blood flow becomes constricted. Just think of it as trying to blow air into a balloon, but the end of the balloon is all stuck together, making it really tough for you to get air through.

If the blood flow is slowed enough or stopped the result is a heart attack or stroke. This is very serious stuff.

What happens is by munching on too many carbohydrates - breads, pastries, tasty sweet snacks, you are stressing your blood sugar levels and forcing them to the extreme. Having high levels of blood sugars will increase your risk of a lipid profile, increases your chances of making heart disease your reality. Studies show that it's not the natural simple sugars that are the issue, but rather the added sugars, the bad ones that are knowingly causing your body harm. This will make your tri-glyceride levels higher will negatively affecting your good and bad cholesterol. Excess sugars are bad news for your heart health.

Osteoporosis
Osteoporosis is a disease that makes your bones weaker and less dense. "Osteo" is bone and "porosis" is porous. Without enough calcium and phosphorus protein is lost, bones thing, break more easily and unfortunately this is a degenerative disease.

Where does sugar fit in with osteoporosis?
You're owner to about 63 TRILLION cells and each one has a brain of its own, so to speak. It's truly amazing how your body is able to manage all of these separate cells and get them to function as one gynormous unit. We are going to take a minute to look a little deeper into integrated function, that importance of stabilizing blood sugars.

POINT ONE - REGULATION BLOOD SUGAR
Inside of you are thousands of automated thermostats. These switches are programmed to raise and lower, turn on and off as required for your body to function. Your "thermostats" take care of water in and outside of each cell, temperatures, hormone regulation, blood health and pressure, blood sugars and so much more.

Let's focus in on your blood sugar levels because they give fuel to your cells and directly affect the function of all your cells every second of every day. Low blood sugar, hypoglycemia and higher blood sugar, diabetes will immediately stress all cells and cause you harm.

Low Blood Sugar . . .
Leaves you feeling tired and sluggish, grumpy and often craving sugary sweets.

High Blood Sugar . . .
Will make you incredibly thirsty and hungry. It can also lead to serious infections and blindness.

Fact is both of these scenarios can be prevented and controlled by paying attention to sugar consumption. In other words preventable, which is where the Sugar Detox fits in.

Obesity-Related Disease
Too much of any food is just not a good thing. Excess sugar over long periods of time will cause health issues for you in the future, eventually anyway. This isn't about going a little crazy once in a while in the sugar department. Perhaps overloaded on chocolate at Easter or indulging with one too many pies during the holidays. Leave the past in the past right where it belongs. This is about today and what you want for your future. Too much sugar is not good for you. So what are you going to do about it?

Excess sugar is going to make you fat and this raises your risk of all sorts of disease and illness, chronic or otherwise. From high blood pressure, diabetes, stroke, kidney and liver disease, to fertility issues, hormone disease, sleep issues, various cancers, bone disease and even mental conditions.

Having a BMI, Body Mass Index over 25, which is high, increases your risk of serious disease. If your BMI is above 30, you're obese and need help ASAP.

My Thoughts . . .
Sugar over consumption is a huge issue today. Doctors and experts are urging society to take action now. There is ample proof that sugar interferes with the smooth function of your bodily system. Making blood flow less than is should, forcing the heart to beat faster, sending moods through a roller coaster ride unnecessarily, fooling around with hormone levels and causing mistiming with other intricate internal systems. Doctors around the world describe long-term sugar consumption as poison. Too much sugar will kill you and the Sugar Detox WILL help. Do I have your attention?

Sugar Detox 101

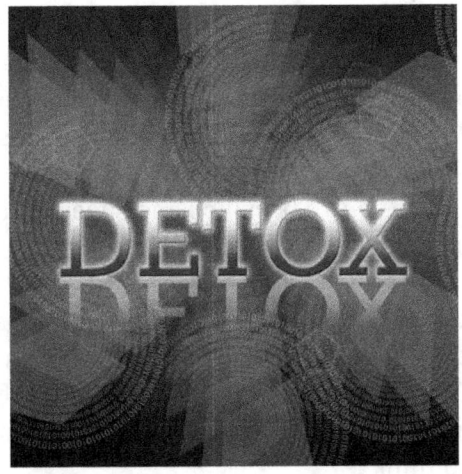

First, we are going to explain what SUGAR ADDICTION is and then the DETOX, just so you understand what you are dealing with.

Small Sugar Addiction - If you've got a small addiction, you are normally dependent on at least one can of pop and perhaps a sweet or two if you want to make it through the day without too much drama. Is this where you fit?

Medium Sugar Addiction - Now if you are making sweets of any sort a dietary requirement with every meal, you have a medium addiction. If you are also dependent on having sweets for snacks religiously you've just put the nail in the wood.

Sugar Bug - Many don't recognize how sugar affects your thinking. Cravings happen when your brain doesn't have enough serotonin, causing a feeling of sadness and low energy. Not enough sugar will make you jittery, moody, quick to blow and give you head pain. Do you have any of these symptoms if you miss a dose of sugar?

Gynormous Sugar Addiction - This is where the large majority of your diet is sugar. It could mean a chocolate bar for breakfast, chips, donuts and pastries for lunch, and maybe a trip to the candy store for a dinner treat. If you grab something sugary every time you turn around and have your purse or car filled with sweets and treats, you are in big trouble, sugar!

What's worse, is if you've been abusing sugar for a long time. Habits are really tough to break as we all know.

Your sugar addiction is mental, physical, emotional and social. This makes it a huge life hurdle. It all comes down to choice. If you want to kick your sugar habit with the Sugar Detox you can. If you don't really want to you won't. Pretty straight forward don't you think?

Sugar is addicting and is in pretty much everything we eat. This also means your actions are negatively affecting your good health.

How-To Sugar Detox
By going on a Sugar Detox you are avoiding sugar and purging it from your system. Sugar is extremely addictive, makes nasty things taste good and yummy things taste better. It's also tough to track exactly how much sugar we feed our body each day. We do know if we've had too much though, because our body will communicate this to us by acting up!

Too much sugar will . . .
* Spike sugar levels, releasing too much insulin, resulting in a sugar rush that eventually lowers energy levels and nutrient absorption.
* Negatively affect your metabolism and cause weight gain.

32

* Turn into blood fat and cholesterol, triggering a melody of health issues.

I'm going to be straight up with you here. Sugar Detox, particularly cold turkey is NOT easy, do-able, but not easy. Mind over matter though and if you truly WANT to change you can and will. No excuses. You control you and if you want it then use the information you learn here, add it to what you already know and will continue learn, and make it happen.

Here are a few strategies to help you successfully implement the Sugar Detox:

Clear Out

If you have sweets and sugary foods within reach, you're going to get into them in weak moments. After all, you're only human. Start by clearing all the sugar out of your house, car, workplace, gym locker and anywhere else you might stash it, hidden stashes too. This is going to help you stay away from sugar and stop triggering it. If you aren't constantly surrounded by sugar and thinking about it, you're less likely to crave it or at least crave is less. It's definitely a step in the right direction.

Time to List ALL Sugar Foods You Eat

It's important you make a list of all the sugar foods you eat and face it. Read this list and go back through your cupboards, workplace, car and all your secret hiding spots and get rid of these foods. This is going to help you break your habit of automatically reaching for cookies in the cupboard when the craving arises, or grabbing a candy bar out of your glove box on the way home from work because you "think" you hungry. Chances are most of it is just pre-programmed by you. Meaning if you have the determination you can reprogram your system to healthy.

Set yourself up for success by slowly reducing the sugary treats you eat. If you normally have a candy bar each afternoon, try

33

having a granola bar instead of just a bite of the candy bar. By slowing reducing the sugar you eat eventually you will see it really isn't necessary and you will eventually get this negative addiction out of your system for good. High sugar foods are recognized as having 37.5-100 grams of sugar per 100 grams of food.

High-Sugar Food List
Beverages
- Fruit juices
- V8 Fusion Vegetable Fruit 100% Juice, Minute Maid Lemonade
- Snapple Iced Tea, vitamin water, instant cocoa

Baked Goods
- Donuts, croissants, cookies
- Muffins,
- Pastries, pies, tarts, squares

Milk Products
- Cream substitute
- Canned, condensed, sweetened milk
- Milkshakes
- Milk, dairy, ice cream
- Instant breakfasts, whipped topping
- Yoplait Thick & Creamy Yogurt
- Weight Watchers Mint Chocolate Chip Ice Cream Cups
- Skinny Cow Ice Cream

Breads and Cereals, Breakfast Foods
- Waffles, Grape nuts cereal
- White bread, white bagels
- Stuffing, shredded wheat, cereal bars, Pop Tarts
- Instant cream of wheat, instant oatmeal, Kellogg's Frosted Mini-Wheat's,
- Ego French Toaster Sticks, Ego Cinnamon Toast Waffles

Snacks
- Jell-o pudding, canned fruit

- Ding Dongs, Twinkies
- Granola bars, Nutri-Grain Bars
- Pretzels, rice cakes, corn chips, potato chips,
- Fruit snacks
- Bran Flakes, Soda crackers

Sauces/Spreads

- Prego 3-Cheese spaghetti sauce, barbecue sauce, ketchup
The idea here is to use common sense and slowly, but surely eliminate these high sugar foods from your diet. You want to shift gears and let the sugar fade out of your everyday and re-place it with healthy, wholesome, nutritional eating. Picking foods below the glycemic index is going to get your body running smoothly without sugar interference and this is something that will make you shine.

FIRST CHOICE - Foods Below Glycemic Index
- Avocados, onions and garlic
- Lettuce, all mixed greens, broccoli, cauliflower, chard, kale, cabbage, Brussels sprouts
- Eggs, fish, chicken, wild game, turkey and pork
- All mushrooms
Next you want to eat foods that are under the low glycemic index.

Low Glycemic Index Foods
- Whole grain breads and bagels
- Whole grain pasta, rice, barley and bulgur
- Chickpeas, kidney beans, baked beans, soy beans, split peas
- Sweet potato, yams
- Oat bran, All Bran and mixed grains
- Cashews, peanuts, almonds, walnuts
- Blackberries, blueberries, strawberries, cherries, kiwi, apples, pears

My Thoughts . . .

Essentially eating healthy will ensure you aren't overloading your system with harmful sugars. Using these lists you can get plenty of healthy fruits and vegetables, lean meats, healthy whole grains and very little milk products. For example cheese in general has few carbohydrates but the little it does have will eventually be converted into sugar and injected into your bloodstream. It's important you are aware of this and depending on your scenario it may or may not be a wise move.

It's all about setting yourself up for success and as your progress over time, as your sugar dependency decreases, you will be able to fine-tune your eating more. With the focus of making sure you are still giving your body all the vitamins and minerals it requires on a regular basis while reducing or removing sugars. Focus on making one change at a time and giving it the duration it requires to become habit. This is how you will success in the Sugar Detox.

Benefits of Sugar Detox

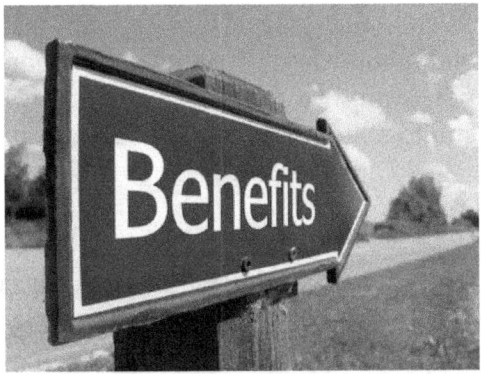

Experts agree that sugar as we consume it today is DEADLY DANGEROUS. Regular Sugar Detox is a wise move and getting rid of sugar for good with a healthy diet change is optimal. Understandably this just doesn't work for some people due to preferences and tolerances and wants, needs and desires.

Most consume far more sugar than required with a heavy reliance on unhealthy snacks and convenience foods that give quick short-term energy boosts. It's not practical in the long-run, but tough to stop because they are so addictive in nature. Simply put the more you eat, the more you crave and want. Here are a few benefits you'll experience from the Sugar Detox.

Lose Weight
Who doesn't want to get rid of fat rolls? One of the first things you'll notice with Sugar Detox is weight loss, a combination of water and fluid loss and fat. The sugar you've been consuming is a tremendous number of extra calories, which just ends up being stored as fat on your thighs, tummy, hips, arms, butt, and any other place it decides to stick. By cutting out all the refined

sugars you're eating you'll cut back loads of fat and calories your body is used to getting. It's inevitable the pounds will just drop off and maybe your pants too!

Bye-Bye Extreme Fatigue
When you sent your energy levels through ups and down all day long depending on when you're injecting your sugar fixes into your bloodstream, you are causing chaos with your energy levels. One minute after a sugar fix you're bouncing off the walls. The next you are depressed and down in the basement, lethargic and ready for a nap.

Getting sugar out of your system will allow your body fluids to stabilize and run toxin-free, smooth as silk with level blood sugars.

Diminished Food Craving
This one will heighten before it fades so be prepared when you're doing the Sugar Detox. As a society we tend to fuel our bodies with cakes, pastries, sweets, coffee shop treats that we eat out of habit, not really because we are hungry or need the nutrition. Most cakes, pastries and high-carb eats lack the vitamins and minerals we need anyway. Regardless we eat them because they look tempting, taste good, and there's usually at least a couple people around you indulging happily.

After a Sugar Detox you will see the cravings for sugar foods will drop considerably. It will take a while for it to completely dissipate, but that's to be expected. It's the same with anything. Fact is the longer you stay away from sugar the less you will crave it. That's just the way the cookie crumbles. You just have to be reasonable here because it will take some time to get all traces out of your system.

Better Energy
Sugar Detox is going to shoot your energy levels straight up. Your system is taxed when you are rocking back and forth with

your energy levels all day long, something sugar does so easily. You are better off to coast through the day on even par, with your energy level and constant. This will make you feel better and give you the consistent energy you need to make it through the day with some still left in your tank.

Thinking Straight
Sugar Detox isn't going to necessarily make you smarter, but it will help you think straighter, which is all good. Experts associate that "fog" thinking or daze that clouds your thinking about sugar. Sugar in excess does interfere with your thought process and if your body is forced to handle more than its fair share you will wind up a little hazy in the think department. Decision making, logic and memory are compromised when your diet is loaded with sugar. This will affect your mood and drive in life. Crystal clear thinking is a sure bet when you get that troublesome sugar gone from your body.

My Thoughts . . .
These rewards from purging your system of sugar are amazing. Until you get it done it really is tough to describe how it's so worth it! Keep in mind doing this Sugar Detox doesn't mean you are never ever in a million years ever going to have sugar again, not unless you want that.

It's perfectly normal to indulge a little with the sweet stuff on special occasions. Just make sure this "time out" is short and sweet. Enjoy it but right after you are done get to a Sugar Detox to get your psychosomatically and physically functioning optimally. You deserve to look and feel great and you will experience this through the benefits of the Sugar Detox.

Side Effects Sugar Detox

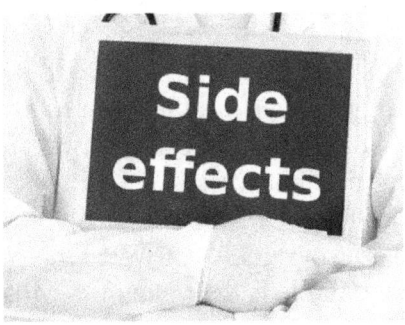

I'd be leading you down the garden path if I didn't at least mention the flip side of the coin. Please keep in mind in the big picture of great health and wellness, these inevitable side effects are like an ant on a mountain, present but hardly noticeable.

Moods Exaggerated

When you make any sort of change in your eating that takes something away, good or bad, that you've been dependent on or are addicted too, you will be moody. Make sure you warn your loved ones, friends and neighbors, so you don't scare them anymore than normal. Excess sugar affects your hormones and chemical balance. When you remove the sugar or even just adjust it your mood can't help, but swing with the chemical shift in your body. You could end up grumpy, easily agitated, impatient and short to blow. Expect this and understand that it's just part of the Sugar Detox process.

Willpower and Perseverance Required

This isn't going to be easy so you might as well swallow that pill straight up. As humans we are resistant to change, find comfort in routine and habit and are masters in talking ourselves out of things that require effort. BE READY to be mentally tough here and work your way through the initial stages of the Sugar Detox.

Chances are your body is very used to getting a nice fix of sugar regularly, loads of carbohydrates, and it will take a strong mind to make it through the initial 3-5 days. Focus on that and understand it will get easier. It's the same sort of thinking as starting an exercise program. The hardest part is starting and the next hardest is the first week.

If you focus and set your goals you WILL do it. Having someone hold you accountable is really helpful. Most have no trouble letting themselves down but it's harder when another person is in the picture.

Extreme Tiredness

You are going to feel extremely lethargic the first few days especially. Gas is being taken suddenly and this will shock your system. Your system is so used to absorbing these sugars induced cyclic ups and downs that are more than likely patterned, it has to be affected when the main ingredient is missing. So, it's reacting to no sugar and it's also working hard to purge all the harmful toxins from your body. Your body is adjusting for the better and you're going to feel tired.

Head Pain

You are unique and the head pain can be in the form of headaches, migraines or even TMJ pain. This pain may be mild or extremely painful. Give yourself time to work through it and make sure you stay hydrated by drinking plenty of water.

My Thoughts . . .
Nobody wants to feel like crap one minute and on top of the world the next. Feeling great all the time is what you should be striving for. Is that going to be your reality? Not likely. Can you get close to that if you eat healthy, exercise and make

smart lifestyle choices? Absolutely. The Sugar Detox is going to help you do just that. These minor and very temporary side effects are well worth it when all is said and done.

Keep in mind everything in life is give and take. If you want to do well on a test you've got to put in the study time. If you want to get to work you've got to pay to put gas in your car. Landing a new job means you've got to have a great resume and interview.

The same things apply if you want to get your body working efficiently and effectively, and if you want to look and feel fabulous. The Sugar Detox will bring you one step closer to a better you. Who wouldn't want that?

Maintenance Plan Pointers

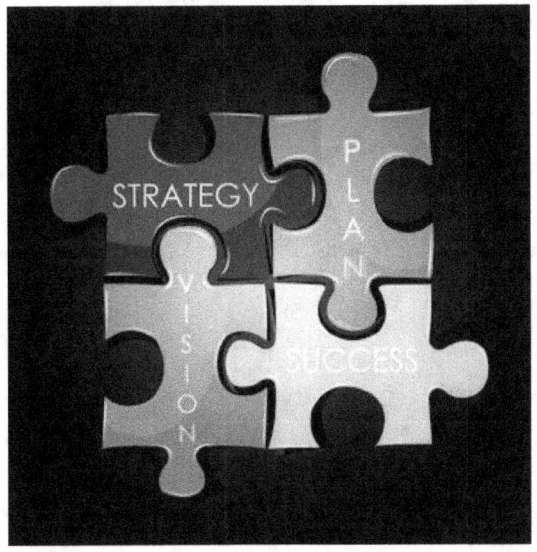

Thank God nobody's perfect! Could you imagine how boring life would be? There would be nothing to work towards and strive for, no goals and aspirations, nothing to change because there is nothing to adjust. Yikes!

On that note it's important you understand how to maintain your healthy lifestyle changes instilled through the Sugar Detox. The last thing you want to do is work hard to eliminate all the toxic sugars from your blood and organs only to dump it all back in just because you haven't thought far enough in advance about maintenance.

Here are a few pointers that are going to help keep you positively focused in life and not on the sugar. When removing sugar from your body you are going to need to replace it, in other words fill the void. Create new habits that aren't going to contribute to health issues and feeling like crap.

* **Take Care of You** - While removing a negative from your life, sugar, fill it with a positive, something for you. By making a point of taking care of yourself you are going to be more open to making the Sugar Detox happen and stick.

Maybe you enjoy hiking or reading. Make the time each day to ensure you fit this into your day for you. This proves to yourself you care and when you feel loved, even self-love, cooperation and a determination to make positive changes just "is."

Instead of going for ice cream Friday afternoon why not go to the spa instead. Maybe you are used to snacking from the vending machines mid-afternoon. How about you read your book or go for a power walk instead? The idea is to do positive things for you that make you feel better about you. Showing yourself you are worth it!

* **Don't Focus Just on Weight Loss** - Yes you are going to lose lots of weight on a Sugar Detox. Although it's important to ensure this isn't your only focus because your weight is going to come off at its own rate and this can become discouraging if your expectations don't like up. Some drop 15-20 pounds in the first couple weeks, stay level for a while and then sporadically lose fat after that. Others start slowly and seem to steadily drop weight. Point is you just don't know and that's why focusing on how you feel and learning what other positive lifestyle changes you can be making is important and productive.

Get into your head this is a long-term move. You want to teach your body to not crave toxic sugar and to adapt a healthy diet that is Sugar Detox based for the most part, allowing exceptions to the rules on special occasions, stamping those exceptions to the rules.

So don't just measure your success on the weight you've dropped. Think about how much clearer your thinking. How you have no more crazy energy shifts and for the most part you are feeling good throughout the day with constant energy. Challenge yourself to come up with other improvements in your life since kissing sugar good-bye. Simply amazing!

* Have a Fan Club - A support system to cheer you on and pick you up when you're down is essential to success. The last think you need in a moment of weakness is people around you urging you to come with them for a devilish dessert feast! Initially, you will need all the help you can get to keep sugar foods out of sight. Out of sight out of mind is practical and it works. Make sure your family doesn't leave sweets and treats around the house. You may want to go so far as having them hide everything from you. Steer clear of baking or going into bakeries or candy stores.

With a little time you will curb your cravings and find that you now have more control. This is something you will always have to work on. Learn about yourself, your weaknesses and life situations where you are more likely to reach for the sweets. The better you know what's in front of you the more prepared you can be. Having full support in this is only going to help you succeed.

* Be Reasonable - You are only human. Expect you are going to take a few steps back before you shift into fifth. So what? Learn to forgive yourself, recognize when you've slipped, and get back on track pronto. Life is all about learning and this includes mucking up from time to time. The important thing here is that you get yourself back on track all eyes forward.

If you had a piece of pumpkin pie at Christmas time, no worries! Make sure you enjoy it and realize it's okay to have a sweet on special occasions. But, it is alright only if you know enough to not go crazy and pick up where you left off the next day. You worked much too hard getting sugar out of your system to throw the towel in completely and start again from scratch. Don't let that happen!

* Learn to Forgive Yourself - Most people associate shame with their sugar addiction. They really can't believe how they let it get out of hand. It's important that you understand the important thing here is that you realized how your sugar addiction was negatively affecting your health. This is a good thing!

Your sugar addiction is not a defect in you. Often it's because of biological reasons, long-learned habits, your environment and social pressures, to start anyway. I'm not saying you can point the blame, but you can chill and realize it's not a flaw in your character that caused your sugar addiction. So there is absolutely nothing wrong with YOU!

Forgive yourself, understand this isn't your fault and be proud you are taking positive action to change it. Just think about all the sickness and heartache you are preventing with Sugar Detox. Not to mention how much more pleasurable and level headed you will be to hang around.

When you release self-blame you will also be able to get rid of sugar once and for all.

* Annual Sugar Detox Weeks - Some people do the Sugar Detox and adopt it for life, looking to shape their everyday eating by keeping sugars out. Others look to completely detox their body, but then find an eating pattern that eliminates sugars for the most part, but not completely. What's important is that regardless of what rhythm you find, it's important to make certain your completely purge your body of sugar on a routine basis. It doesn't matter whether this is once a month, once or twice a year. Every single time you lower or eliminate the sugars in your internal systems you are doing your body and mind a favor.

Never forget this and you will always be inching your way towards a brighter, energized and happier you.

My Thinking . . .
Most diet and lifestyle changes fail because we fail to think about long-term maintenance. Sure we might hit our initial goals, but we don't understand how to incorporate our new healthy habits into our life for life. Think this through and use these pointers to set yourself up for success with the Sugar Detox. Open your mind and make sure you have a plan. That's exactly what you need.

Sugar Myths/Truths

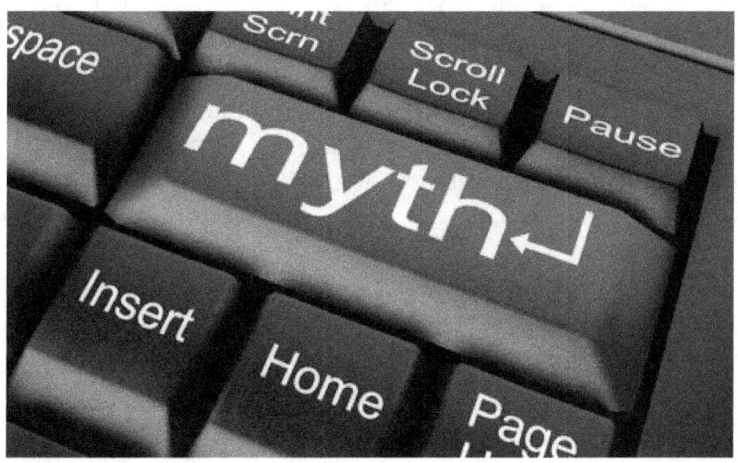

You can't handle the truth! Or can you? There are always mis-truths around that screw around with our perception. Having the facts from which to build is only going to help you take more effective action in whatever you are doing. If you were a runner and thought that running on the pavement is best, eventually after developing ruined knees and hips you would figure out that sort of running is the worst. If you had the truth from the get-go, that cushioned running, like on sand or a softer surface with very good running shoes is best, you would still be running today.

Same thing applies with sugar. Understanding which statements are truthful and which aren't is important if making the best decisions for you. Here are a few sugar myths I'd like to clear up to ensure you've got the "right" information to better you.

Myth One - Sugar Makes You Fat
Truth: Sugar is found naturally and a substance your body
needs to get healthy. Fruits and vegetables have natural or simple sugars for instance and healthy, loaded with vitamins,
minerals and essential fiber. The problem arises when we consume too much sugar, a huge issues in society today.
Many foods we eat are not natural and loaded with extra fat
and sugar. Fast food restaurants, vending machines, convenience stores and bakeries come to mind. Places we frequent
that serve nothing but, sugar. Fat and sugar that in time will
make us fat.

Myth Two - Eating Sugar Will Make Children Hyper
Truth: Some children act hyper when they have a sudden
surge in blood sugar levels. The glycemic index measures this,
the amount of sugar in a particular food. The higher the number, the quicker the conversion is to blood sugar. Studies show
that sugar does not affect the thinking and behavior of most
normal children, although there may be a select group of children that are more sensitive to sugar than others.

Myth Three - By Eating Healthy You Get Rid Of All Sugar
Truth: Sugar is a natural element and would be impossible to
eliminate all sugar from your diet, not if you wanted to eat to
survive and be healthy. The only food it isn't found in naturally
is meat and good luck surviving on meat and nothing else.
It's the added sugars that do your body harm you want to get
rid of. The refined sugars and sweeteners are the culprits that
interfere with your good health, steal your energy, cloud your
thinking, stress your internal systems and increase your risk for
serious disease to start. Just regards to sugar.

Myth Four - Consuming Sugar Will Cause Diabetes
Truth: Diabetes is a result of the body not producing enough
insulin or the cells not responding to the insulin produced. The
function of insulin is to regulate blood sugars and when this
isn't working the blood sugar levels shoot through the roof as

too much insulin is produced. Type 1 diabetes is mainly genetic. Type 2 diabetes is a result of genetics and an unhealthy lifestyle. Often it's linked to obesity, high fat eating and little or no exercise. So indirectly sugar is connected with the development of diabetes, guilty by associated, although it isn't the cause of it.

Myth Five - White Sugar is the Worst For You
Truth: White sugar is no worse for you than brown, powdered, or corn syrup. Refined sugars in general are bad for your body and your thinking. Opting to switch them for natural sugars is the right move. When comparing the two sugars natural sugars take longer to break down than refined sugars, providing energy longer, they also contain more nutrients than your refined option.

Myth Six - Eating Sugar is Going to Make you Wrinkle
Truth: Recent studies found that damaged proteins are linked with early aging and sugar is linked with harming these proteins. However it was later discovered the damage was caused by sugars, complex carbohydrates, protein and fats. Bottom line is sugar doesn't make you crinkle.

My Thoughts . . .
Getting to the bottom of these sugar myths will help fuel you with positive and factual information to help you understand sugar better and make the smooth adjustment to eliminating it from your diet. Knowing the truth is the first step in making a solid plan to move you one step closer to better health and happiness. Onward!

Sugar Tidbit - Artificial Sweeteners Explained
Sweeteners are used to replace natural sugars. You will find them in low-calorie beverages and foods. You may have heard to them referred to as "empty" calories.

People substitute various artificial sweeteners into their coffee or tea, they can be used in baking to cut calories, people even use artificial sweeteners to add more sweetness to strawberries and fresh fruit.

Diet sodas have zero calories because of artificial sweeteners instead of natural sugars.

Artificial sweeteners and Diet go hand in hand.

The six unhealthy artificial sweeteners approved for use by the Health and Food Administration are: Neotame, Saccharin, Aspartame, Acesulfame, Sucralose, and Potassium.

You've probably heard of Aspartame and Sucralose most often, they're considered the most dangerous.

Sucralose is fairly new to our markets and falls under the name Splenda. Essentially it's sugar that's chemically altered by taking out three hydroxyl groups and adding three chlorine atoms. In case you weren't aware, chlorine does cause cancer. This artificial sweetener was approved because there are no long-term studies to prove it kills. People are going to have to get sick and die before it's taken off the shelves.

Aspartame is sold under NutraSweet or Equate. Literally thousands of products contain aspartame. Sodas, jell-o, pudding, gum, and yogurts are a few common items with this artificial sweeteners. Unfortunately money trumps everything. Very powerful people got a hold of it and approved it to go on the grocery shelves. Regardless of the fact there are lots of scientific studies claiming birth defects, epilepsy, brain tumors, diabetes, and mental retardation to start. Unfortunately no moves have been made to get rid of it yet.

Conclusion

The Sugar Detox is something everyone will benefit from, regardless of your age, lifestyle, nutrition knowledge or walk of life. Prevention is the key in preserving your quality of life and ensuring you are happier longer.

By taking control of your health you are able to take control of your life and implement strategies to improve it. Sugar destroys teeth, fools with hormone levels, triggers bouts of fatigue, is a causal factor in various cancers and serious disease, contributes to obesity and directly clouds your thinking.

Sugar interferes with you mentally and physically, increasing stress and this too will eventually take its toll. The Sugar Detox will challenge you positively. It won't be easy, but the rewards of removing this toxic substance from your system will make it more than worth it. What's not to love about thinking with clarity, feeling energetic and alive, getting rid of self-created energy highs and lows, and deterring serious disease and illness?

The ball is in your court my friend. Take a shot! You've got nothing to lose and better health and wellness to gain.

We have the choice to look for the positive or the negative in life. You can choose to lift someone up or to stomp on them. Writing is my passion and I work hard at it, with the goal of helping make people better. If you gain a new piece of knowledge, read something that makes you think, or perhaps even smile a few times, then I am happy and content!

Life's just too short not to tune into optimism. If your glass is half full, then I invite you to read my writing, and if you have a minute to spare when you're through, **I would appreciate your review.** This will help me better myself and my writing. I thank you in advance and appreciate you.